UNDERSTANDING

L-THEANINE

AND BENEFITS

A Guide To Uncover Its Targets, Focus On Cognitive Advantages, And Embrace A Healthier Lifestyle Through In-Depth Knowledge And Application

DR. LACEY MICHELLE

Disclaimer:

The information provided in this book is for general informational purposes only and is not intended as medical advice.

Readers are encouraged to consult with a qualified healthcare professional for any health concerns or questions.

The author of this book is not affiliated with any individual, website, organization, or products mentioned within.

This book does not endorse or promote any specific brands, services, or external entities. Any references made are purely for illustrative purposes and should not be construed as endorsements.

Readers are responsible for their own decisions and should conduct their own research before making any health-related choices.

Any liability resulting from the use of this information, whether direct or indirect, is disclaimed by the author and publisher.

Contents

CHAPTER ONE...................................12

An Overview Of L-Theanine: 12

History And Discovery: 13

Natural L-Theanine Sources:................14

Chemical Composition And Characteristics
....15

How The Body Reacts To L-Theanine.....17

Systems Of Action.............................18

CHAPTER TWO 22

Advantages Of L-Theanine For Health......22

Improving Cognitive Function 23

Slumber And Leisure 24

Heart-Related Health 26

Immune System Assistance................27

CHAPTER THREE..............................30

Caffeine With L-Theanine: An Intriguing Pair
....30

The Benefits Of L-Theanine And Caffeine
Together.......................................30

Increased Alertness And Focus............32

Striking The Correct Balance...............33

CHAPTER FOUR 36

Safety And Dosage Of L-Theanine..........36

Suggested Rationales 36

Possible Adverse Reactions.................37

Interactions Between Drugs.................38

Safety & Safety Measures....................39

CHAPTER FIVE 42

Choosing Supplements With L-Theanine ..42

Variations In L-Theanine Forms...........42

Choosing An Excellent Supplement 44

Options And Forms Of Dosage.............46

CHAPTER SIX....................................48

Including L-Theanine In Your Daily Routine:
....48

Choosing The Best L-Theanine Product:.49

Useful Advice For Everyday Use: 50

CHAPTER SEVEN 52

L-Theanine In Combination With Other
Supplements: 52

Speak With A Healthcare Professional: ..53

How To Include L-Theanine In Your Diet:
....54

CHAPTER EIGHT 58

Research On L-Theanine And Its Prospects
....58

New Research Fields:............................59

Potential Future Uses:...........................61

Testimonies And First-Hand Accounts....63

Applications In The Real World And
Success Stories....................................65

Professional Responses And Explanations
....69

Conclusion..71

About This Book:

Explores the complex world of L-Theanine, including its pharmacological underpinnings, historical origins, and several health advantages. This thorough reference, designed for both health lovers and inquisitive minds, takes readers on a tour through the history, purposes, and real-world uses of L-theanine.

Synopsis of Leucine

Historical Context

Objective and Range of the Book

Intended Readership

Knowledge of L-Theanine

L-theanine: What is it?

Where to Find L-Theanine

Properties and Structure of Chemicals

Mechanisms at Work

Metabolism and Absorption

Advantages of L-Theanine for Health

Reduction of Stress and Anxiety

Improving Intelligence

Improvement of Sleep

Support for the Immune System

Health of the Heart

Antioxidant Characteristics

L-Theanine and Emotional Wellbeing

Effect on Endocrine Systems

Connection to Serotonin and Dopamine

Possibility of Treating Mood Disorders

Attention and Cognitive Processes

Useful Applications

Suggested Doses

Optimal Guidelines for Ingestion

Possible Adverse Reactions and Safety Measures

Relationships with Other Drugs

Investigations and Scholarly Research

Synopsis of Clinical Research

Major Discoveries and Outcomes

Remarks and Restrictions

Prospective Paths of Research

L-Theanine in Different Contexts

Vitamins & Supplements

Tea's L-Theanine

Nutritional Sources

Comparing Various Formats

Customer Viewpoints

User Reviewed Content

Triumphant Accounts

Difficulties and Cons

Aspects Related to Regulation

Legal Position

Safety Guidelines

Quality Assurance

In summary

Describe L-theanine.

CHAPTER ONE

An Overview Of L-Theanine:

Mostly present in tea leaves, especially in green tea (Camellia sinensis), L-Theanine is an amino acid. It is well recognized for its possible relaxing and cognitive-enhancing benefits and is frequently taken as a dietary supplement. Because it can penetrate the blood-brain barrier and affect the central nervous system, L-theanine is a special kind of chemical. Although it shares structural similarities with the excitatory neurotransmitter glutamate, its functions in the brain are very distinct. L-theanine is a well-liked option for people trying to lower their stress and anxiety levels because it is thought to encourage relaxation without making you sleepy.

History And Discovery:

In 1949, Japanese scientists working under the direction of Dr. Takeshi Hirayama made the initial discovery of L-theanine while examining the chemical makeup of tea leaves. Because of its occurrence in tea, the compound was originally referred to as "theine."

However, more research showed that the compound's molecular structure was identical to that of L-Theanine. It was discovered that this amino acid was in charge of giving green tea its distinct umami flavor.

The growing body of research on L-Theanine's possible health benefits throughout time has made it a popular dietary supplement.

Natural L-Theanine Sources:

Tea is the main natural source of L-Theanine, with green tea having the highest concentration. L-theanine is an amino acid that is plentiful in green tea, although other tea varieties, such as black and white tea, also include it.

The same plant that yields tea leaves, Camellia sinensis, contains L-theanine in its leaves. L-theanine is commonly consumed in tea-drinking countries such as China and Japan, partly due to its natural source.

It is thought to have a role in the relaxing and alerting effects of tea consumption. Apart from tea, a few edible mushrooms also contain trace levels of L-theanine, although at far lower concentrations than in tea leaves.

L-theanine has also been made available as a supplement in recent years as a result of growing interest in its possible health advantages.

For people looking for L-Theanine's particular properties, these supplements are frequently utilized to deliver a concentrated and standardized amount of the drug. L-theanine, whether it comes from tea or supplements, is still being studied by scientists because of its possible effects on several areas related to human health and well-being.

Chemical Composition And Characteristics

L-theanine, or just theanine, is an amino acid that is mostly present in tea leaves, namely those of the Camellia sinensis plant, which is the source of tea.

It shares structural similarities with the neurotransmitters glutamine and glutamate in the brain.

L-theanine differs from other amino acids in that its chemical structure is a special mixture of an amine group and an ethyl ester group. Its biological activity and interaction with the human body depend on this structural characteristic.

Unlike other amino acids, L-theanine is not used in the formation of proteins, making it a non-protein amino acid. Rather, it is well-known for its psychotropic qualities, most notably its capacity to provide calm without sedation.

Because of its unique chemical makeup, it can cross the blood-brain barrier and influence brain activity in addition to having a range of cognitive and psychological effects on the body.

How The Body Reacts To L-Theanine

L-theanine works mainly in the brain via interacting with neurotransmitters, namely by adjusting the activity of glutamate, dopamine, and gamma-aminobutyric acid (GABA). Its ability to raise alpha brain wave activity—which is connected to a state of calm awareness—is one of its most notable properties. During meditation, daydreaming, and times of wakeful relaxation, alpha brain waves are frequently seen.

L-theanine's impact on GABA receptors is responsible for its capacity to induce calm and lessen anxiety. In the brain, GABA functions as an inhibitory neurotransmitter, assisting in the regulation of excitatory neurotransmitters such as glutamate. L-theanine has a relaxing and anxiolytic effect because it increases GABA synthesis and receptor sensitivity. L-theanine's ability to lower stress and elevate mood is attributed to this mechanism.

Additionally, L-theanine can influence the release and control of other neurotransmitters. It has been demonstrated to enhance dopamine release, a neurotransmitter linked to motivation and pleasure. L-theanine may help with focus and a better sense of well-being by affecting dopamine levels.

Systems Of Action

L-theanine's distinctive effects on mood and cognitive function are the result of a complex interaction of biochemical processes in the body, which are the mechanism of action.

The following are some of the main ways that L-theanine works:

Glutamate Modulation: By preventing glutamate from binding to specific receptors, L-theanine can control the amount of this excitatory neurotransmitter released. In doing so, it promotes a calmer mental state and helps avoid excessive neuronal activation.

GABA Enhancement: L-theanine raises the sensitivity of GABA receptors and increases the synthesis of GABA, an inhibitory neurotransmitter.

This lowers anxiety, encourages relaxation, and might even improve the quality of your sleep.

Alpha Brain Wave Activation: Relaxation, enhanced focus, and a decrease in stress are linked to L-theanine's capacity to enhance alpha brain wave activity.

Neurotransmitter Release: L-theanine can improve mood, motivation, and general cognitive performance by affecting dopamine release and reuptake.

Blood-Brain Barrier Penetration: Because of its special structure, L-theanine can pass across the blood-brain barrier and directly interact with neurotransmitters and brain receptors.

L-theanine's physiological impacts on the body and mind are numerous, and its significance as an intriguing amino acid is further highlighted by the science behind it.

Its reputation as an effective supplement for encouraging relaxation, lowering stress levels, and improving cognitive function is partly due to its chemical makeup, ability to influence neurotransmitters, and effect on brain wave activity.

Scholars investigating the possible medicinal uses of this organic substance are nevertheless intrigued by the many ways in which L-theanine functions.

CHAPTER TWO

Advantages Of L-Theanine For Health

Reducing Stress and Managing Anxiety

The amino acid L-theanine, which is mostly present in tea leaves, is becoming known for its ability to encourage relaxation and lessen tension and anxiety.

It has a reputation for relaxing the nervous system without making people feel sleepy. L-theanine functions by boosting the synthesis of many neurotransmitters that are involved in mood regulation, including dopamine and serotonin.

This makes it an effective tool for stress and anxiety management since it enables people to remain composed and cool in the face of everyday obstacles.

Studies have indicated that L-theanine can produce a state of alert relaxation by regulating alpha brain waves, which has a calming effect on the brain.

It is well known that the molecule lessens the physiological reactions to stress, including elevated blood pressure and heart rate, which are usually connected to the "fight or flight" response.

Because of this, L-Theanine is widely used as a natural, non-sedating substitute for prescription drugs in the treatment of stress and anxiety.

Improving Cognitive Function

L-theanine has demonstrated potential in augmenting cognitive function and elevating focus and attention in addition to its anxiolytic effects. L-theanine, which is naturally present in tea, when combined with caffeine can help reduce the jitters and anxiety that are frequently brought on by caffeine intake while also fostering improved mental clarity. L-theanine and caffeine work in concert to enhance cognitive clarity and task performance.

The benefits of L-theanine on cognition are thought to be related to its effects on neurotransmitters, namely raising the levels of GABA (gamma-aminobutyric acid), an amino acid that has inhibitory effects on brain activity. L-theanine promotes a healthy balance between alertness and relaxation, which helps people retain mental clarity and improves their capacity to deal with difficult situations and obstacles.

Slumber And Leisure

The ability of L-theanine to promote relaxation without sedation also suggests that it may enhance the quality of one's sleep. It may be especially helpful for people who have trouble falling asleep or have insomnia because it promotes serenity and reduces anxiety.

The substance can regulate the circadian rhythm, promoting a more seamless descent into slumber and enhancing restorative sleep in general.

Additionally, by extending the length of deep, slow-wave sleep—which is crucial for both physical and mental renewal—L-theanine may improve the quality of sleep. Because it lowers stress and improves the quality of sleep, L-Theanine is a useful supplement for people looking for all-natural solutions for sleep-related problems.

Research has been done on the possible cardiovascular advantages of L-theanine. It has demonstrated the capacity to lower blood pressure, which is important for people who have high blood pressure or who are at risk of developing heart-related issues.

By encouraging blood vessel relaxation and lowering the constriction linked to high blood pressure, the substance affects the cardiovascular system.

Moreover, the antioxidant and anti-inflammatory qualities of L-theanine can support general heart health by shielding the circulatory system from oxidative stress and inflammation.

L-theanine, when incorporated into a heart-healthy lifestyle, may provide an additional means of preserving normal cardiovascular function, even though it shouldn't be used as a primary treatment for cardiovascular diseases.

Immune System Assistance

L-theanine may help to boost the immune system, according to research.

It has been demonstrated to increase the generation of immune cells involved in the immunological response, such as gamma delta T cells.

L-theanine may improve an individual's resistance to infections and help them maintain their general health by strengthening the immune system's defense against microorganisms.

L-theanine has anti-inflammatory and stress-relieving qualities that can help the immune system indirectly in addition to actively supporting it.

The body's defenses can be weakened by ongoing stress and inflammation, leaving it more vulnerable to disease.

L-theanine can help sustain a strong and responsive immune system by reducing these adverse effects, particularly in times of increased stress or vulnerability.

To sum up, L-theanine is a flexible supplement that may offer several health advantages.

This amino acid provides a comprehensive approach to well-being, supporting people in maintaining their physical and mental health in a variety of ways.

These benefits range from stress reduction and anxiety management to cognitive enhancement, better sleep, cardiovascular health, and immune system support.

Before beginning any supplementation program, you should speak with a healthcare provider to be sure it is suitable for your unique needs and situation.

CHAPTER THREE

Caffeine With L-Theanine: An Intriguing Pair

There's a solid reason why the pairing of L-theanine with caffeine has been very popular recently. This dynamic pair, which is frequently present in a variety of supplements and drinks, provides a special synergy that may significantly improve general well-being and cognitive function. We'll talk about the research underlying this collaboration and how it improves mental clarity, attentiveness, and focus.

The Benefits Of L-Theanine And Caffeine Together

The way that L-theanine and caffeine interact when taken together is one of their most fascinating features. An instant boost of energy and alertness can be obtained from caffeine, a well-known stimulant that can be found in coffee, tea, and energy drinks. On the other hand, it is also well known for producing jitters and, occasionally, a "crash" after its effects wear off.

Conversely, the amino acid L-theanine is found naturally in tea leaves, especially in green tea. It is well renowned for having calming and soothing qualities.

There's an interesting interaction that happens when you combine L-theanine with caffeine.

L-theanine is remarkably effective in reducing the negative effects of caffeine, like restlessness and anxiety, while boosting its benefits, like increased energy and focus. Achieving the best possible cognitive performance requires striking this equilibrium.

Increased Alertness And Focus

The apparent increase in attention and alertness is the main reason people look for L-theanine plus caffeine supplements or select beverages that have this combination. Caffeine's overstimulating effects are countered by L-theanine, which encourages a relaxed wakefulness.

This implies that one can keep a clear and composed head rather than getting the usual jitters brought on by coffee.

It is believed that the combination of L-theanine and caffeine causes a rise in the release of several neurotransmitters linked to mood and attention modulation, including serotonin and dopamine.

Together, these two may also increase the generation of alpha brain waves, which are linked to relaxed alertness and imaginative thought.

Studies indicate that the combination of L-theanine and caffeine may result in higher problem-solving abilities, quicker reaction times, and better cognitive function.

Furthermore, this combination might support people in maintaining their motivation and concentration for extended periods, which is advantageous for jobs requiring constant attention.

Striking The Correct Balance

It takes skill to find the ideal ratio between L-theanine and caffeine.

The optimal ratio can differ based on a person's unique caffeine sensitivity.

While some people may choose a more balanced strategy to retain a productive mood without excessive stimulation, others may prefer a higher L-Theanine to caffeine ratio for a more relaxing impact.

It's crucial to remember that caffeine and L-theanine aren't just found in energy beverages and supplements.

Many people would rather obtain these components naturally, like in green tea. People can customize their experience to fit their requirements and tastes by experimenting with different ratios and sources.

Caffeine and L-theanine are a powerful illustration of the synergy that can occur between various substances.

Together, they provide a special and potent cognitive improvement tool that promotes increased mental clarity, attention, and alertness.

This dynamic pair may be able to assist people in striking the correct balance between leisure and work, which will eventually improve their general well-being and performance in a variety of spheres of life.

CHAPTER FOUR

Safety And Dosage Of L-Theanine

Natural amino acids like L-theanine can be found in tea leaves, especially in green tea. Because of its possible ability to promote relaxation and reduce tension, it has become more and more popular as a dietary supplement.

The suggested L-theanine dosage varies based on the individual and the desired purpose of the supplement. Typically, a dose should not exceed 400 mg per day. It's crucial to remember that each individual may require a different dosage.

Suggested Rationales

An individual's age, weight, and the purpose of taking the supplement can all affect the recommended dosage of L-theanine. One or two daily doses of 100 to 200 mg are commonly recommended for inducing relaxation and lowering tension. A dosage between 200 and 400 milligrams would be more appropriate for people looking to enhance their focus or cognitive function. It's critical to identify the dose that works best for you by gradually increasing it from a lower starting point. The ideal L-theanine dosage can be found by speaking with a trained nutritionist or healthcare provider, depending on your individual needs and medical conditions.

Possible Adverse Reactions

When used by authorized dosages, L-theanine is generally regarded as safe. Adverse effects are infrequent, and it is well tolerated. On the other hand, some people might have modest adverse effects, such as headaches, lightheadedness, or stomach pain. These negative effects typically subside on their own and are moderate and transient. Different from other supplements or pharmaceuticals used for stress reduction, L-theanine induces relaxation without sedation, thus it usually doesn't make you feel sleepy.

Interactions Between Drugs

While taking L-theanine by itself is generally safe, it's important to think about possible interactions with any other medications or supplements you may be taking. The slight relaxing effects of L-theanine may intensify the sedative qualities of medications such as benzodiazepines, hypnotics, or other CNS-affecting agents.

It's best to speak with a healthcare provider before adding L-Theanine to your regimen if you are taking any prescription medications, especially if they may affect your mental health or cognitive performance. This will help to ensure that there are no negative interactions.

When used properly, most individuals consider L-theanine to be safe. But there are a few things to be aware of and safeguards to take.

There is little data on the safety of L-theanine supplements in pregnant or nursing women, so before taking any, speak with your doctor. Before beginning an L-theanine supplement, anyone with underlying medical conditions—especially those affecting the liver or kidneys—should also consult a physician. L-theanine should always be purchased from reliable vendors to guarantee product quality and purity.

When used at recommended quantities, L-theanine is a typically safe and well-tolerated supplement. It may be advantageous for relieving stress, improving cognitive function, and relaxing.

But just like with any dietary supplement, it's important to be aware of individual differences in reaction, possible drug interactions, and particular health issues.

When in doubt, it's best to speak with a healthcare provider to find out how much L-theanine is right for you and make sure using it will help you achieve your overall wellness and health objectives.

CHAPTER FIVE

Choosing Supplements With L-Theanine

Making educated decisions is essential when thinking about using L-theanine supplements to make sure you're getting the ideal product for your needs. An amino acid called L-theanine is naturally present in tea leaves, particularly in green tea, and is well-known for its capacity to promote calm and reduce stress. It's critical to comprehend the many forms of L-Theanine, how to choose a high-quality supplement, and the range of dosage forms and options accessible before purchasing an L-Theanine supplement.

Variations In L-Theanine Forms

There are various types of L-theanine, each with unique properties and possible benefits. Suntheanine and L-theanine are the two main types. While Suntheanine is a proprietary type of L-Theanine that has undergone a special manufacturing procedure to enhance its purity and consistency, L-Theanine is the natural form found in tea leaves. The decision between these kinds may be based on personal preferences and particular health objectives.

Since L-Theanine is isolated straight from tea leaves and contains additional health-promoting ingredients, some people might prefer this method.

Conversely, suntheanine is frequently preferred due to its purity and lack of impurities. In the end, while selecting a supplement, it's critical to take the source and processing of the L-Theanine into account.

It is crucial to choose a premium L-theanine supplement to guarantee both its effectiveness and safety. To do this, it's wise to take into account the following elements:

Purity: Seek goods that offer comprehensive details regarding the L-Theanine's purity. The percentage of L-Theanine in each serving should be indicated on the label together with the purity level.

Third-party testing: To ensure the purity and potency of your supplements, look for ones that have undergone independent testing. These tests can confirm that the product is free of contaminants and fulfills the claims made on the label.

Ingredients: Check the product's ingredient list to make sure no extraneous allergies, fillers, or additions are included. Supplements of the highest caliber usually contain very few extra ingredients.

Manufacturer reputation: Find out about the reputation of the manufacturer and think about going with well-known, respectable brands that have a track record of manufacturing high-quality supplements.

User reviews: Perusing user reviews and testimonials might offer insightful information about previous customers' experiences using the product, assisting you in making a well-informed choice.

Certifications: Certain supplements may bear certificates indicating quality and safety, such as Certified Organic or Good Manufacturing Practices (GMP).

Options And Forms Of Dosage

L-theanine supplements are available in a range of dose forms and alternatives to accommodate a variety of needs and preferences.

Typical forms include powder, tablets, capsules, and even drinks with L-theanine added. Several considerations, including taste preferences, simplicity of usage, and the intended rate of absorption, can influence the dosage form selection.

For people who would rather have a dose that is already calculated, capsules and tablets are practical choices. They are a well-liked option for use when traveling because they are portable and simple to eat. L-theanine powder offers greater dosing flexibility based on personal needs, however, it might need to be mixed with a beverage.

L-Theanine-infused drinks, such as some teas or relaxation drinks, also provide a tasty option to take in the supplement while still tasting good.

However the amount of L-Theanine in these drinks could differ, so it's important to read the label to find out the precise dosage.

Choosing the best L-Theanine supplement requires researching the many dosage forms and possibilities available, taking into account the varied types of L-Theanine, and settling on a high-quality product.

People can maximize the potential advantages of L-theanine for stress relief and relaxation in their daily lives by making educated decisions.

CHAPTER SIX

Including L-Theanine In Your Daily Routine:

Tea leaves naturally contain an amino acid called L-theanine, which has been shown to have the ability to ease tension and encourage relaxation.

It's critical to comprehend the advantages of L-theanine and how to integrate it into your daily routine. For people looking for a non-prescription solution for stress reduction and cognitive enhancement, this substance may be especially helpful.

L-theanine benefits: L-theanine is well-known for its capacity to promote relaxation without making one feel sleepy. It accomplishes this by encouraging the synthesis of neurotransmitters that are essential for mood control, including serotonin and dopamine.

Moreover, L-theanine is a desirable supplement for people who want to increase their mental clarity because it may enhance cognitive function, such as focus and attention.

Choosing The Best L-Theanine Product: It's critical to choose a reliable and high-quality product when introducing L-Theanine into your lifestyle.

Seek supplements with standardized L-Theanine content that are made from green tea extract. Make sure the product satisfies your dietary requirements—vegan or vegetarian options, for example—and is free of toxins.

dose & Timing: Although individual recommendations for L-theanine dose range from 100 to 400 mg daily, there are certain exceptions. Gradually raise the dosage from a lower starting point as needed. You can take L-theanine with or without food, and when is the best to take it will mostly rely on what you hope to achieve. It may be more beneficial to take it in the evening for relaxation and stress reduction, and in the morning for increased attention.

Useful Advice For Everyday Use:
With a few helpful pointers, adding L-theanine to your daily regimen can be simple.

To get the most out of this supplement, consider the following suggestions:

It's imperative to take L-theanine consistently if you want to reap its full benefits. It could take some time to see results, so be patient and include it in your regular regimen.

Try Different Doses: Everyone reacts differently to L-theanine, so experiment with dosage. Try out various dosages to determine which one works best for you. If necessary, gradually raise the dose from a lower starting point.

Pair with Caffeine: If you like to drink tea or coffee, you might want to think about combining L-theanine with caffeine. The jittery effects that are sometimes linked to caffeine alone might be lessened with this combination, which can offer a balanced and targeted energy increase.

Track Your Stress Levels: To determine how L-theanine affects your well-being, monitor your stress levels and mood. You can assess whether the supplement is beneficial for you by using this self-awareness.

CHAPTER SEVEN

L-Theanine In Combination With Other Supplements:

L-theanine is a useful supplement to have in your regimen; to maximize its benefits or target particular health issues, it is frequently taken in combination with other ingredients.

Synergy with Caffeine: As previously shown, a common combination is L-theanine and caffeine. The combination of these two substances might lessen the possible adverse effects of coffee, such as jitters and anxiety, while simultaneously enhancing alertness, attention, and cognitive function.

Support for Stress and Sleep: L-theanine can be taken in conjunction with other supplements like melatonin, ashwagandha, or valerian root which are said to help with stress or sleep. You can customize these combinations to meet your own needs, be they relaxation or higher-quality sleep.

Nootropic Stacks: L-Theanine is frequently combined with other substances that improve cognition, such as choline sources or racetams, in nootropic stacks. The purpose of these combinations is to enhance general cognitive function, memory, and focus.

Speak With A Healthcare Professional:

It is advisable to speak with a healthcare professional before taking L-theanine in combination with other supplements, particularly if you are on prescription medication or have any underlying medical conditions. They may offer advice and guarantee the efficacy and safety of your supplement plan.

How To Include L-Theanine In Your Diet: In addition to consuming L-Theanine as a supplement, you can include it in your diet by consuming specific foods and beverages.

Drinking Tea:

 Tea leaves naturally contain L-theanine, which is more abundant in green tea. One pleasant and soothing approach to up your L-theanine intake is to drink green tea. Green tea powder, or matcha, is an additional great source.

Dietary Supplements: L-theanine is a component in certain dietary supplements and beverages that promote relaxation.

 For a simple approach to incorporate L-Theanine into your diet, look for these products at health food stores or online.

Try Different Recipes: Use your imagination while preparing meals by experimenting with items high in L-theanine. Try preparing meals with green tea or look into recipes that have tea characteristics.

Balance Your Diet: It's important to keep a balanced diet that contains various nutrients that are necessary for both physical and mental well-being in addition to specialized L-theanine sources.

 Whole grains, fruits, and vegetables are nutrient-rich foods that can enhance the effects of L-theanine.

L-theanine can be incorporated into your lifestyle for several advantages, including reduced stress and enhanced cognitive performance. You may maximize the benefits of this adaptable amino acid by paying attention to its combination with other supplements, experimenting with dosage, and according to some helpful guidelines. Adding a delicious layer to your general well-being can also come from incorporating L-Theanine into your diet through creative cooking or tea use.

To ensure safety and efficacy, don't forget to speak with a healthcare provider before making any major changes to your supplement routine.

CHAPTER EIGHT

Research On L-Theanine And Its Prospects

Current Scientific Research and Conclusions: Because of its possible health advantages and capacity to improve cognitive function, the amino acid L-theanine, which is mostly found in tea leaves, has attracted a lot of attention from scientists.

Several investigations have been carried out to examine its methods of action and effects on human health. According to recent studies, L-theanine may be able to pass through the blood-brain barrier and influence the central nervous system there.

It has been linked to lowering stress and anxiety as well as elevating mood by raising the levels of specific neurotransmitters including dopamine and serotonin. L-theanine is also a topic of interest for people looking to increase focus and concentration because it has shown the ability to boost cognitive function and attention.

L-theanine may also have neuroprotective qualities, which could lessen the impacts of neurodegenerative illnesses and age-related cognitive decline, according to research on the supplement.

Research on its antioxidant qualities has also revealed how it helps the body by lowering inflammation and oxidative stress. As a result, it has been connected to several health advantages, such as enhancing immunological and cardiovascular health.

New Research Fields:

As our understanding of L-theanine deepens, new research fields are illuminating its possible therapeutic uses as well as its mechanisms of action. The relationship between L-theanine and other substances, especially caffeine, is one noteworthy topic of research interest. The exact mechanism by which the relaxing and anxiety-reducing benefits of L-theanine interact with the stimulating effects of caffeine to produce a targeted and well-balanced cognitive boost is still being investigated.

 L-theanine and caffeine supplements have been developed as a result of this combination to enhance cognitive performance.

Moreover, current research has turned its attention to the connection between L-theanine and sleep. According to certain research, L-theanine may be able to provide a natural substitute for pharmaceutical sleep aids by encouraging relaxation and lowering anxiety. Furthermore, research on the impact of L-theanine on mood disorders like bipolar disorder and depression is picking up steam. Scholars are investigating the potential therapeutic advantages of L-theanine on neurotransmitter levels in various illnesses.

Potential Future Uses:

There are a plethora of potential uses for L-theanine research in the future. Its possible application in the treatment of illnesses associated with stress and anxiety is one area of particular attention.

Because it can promote relaxation without sedation, L-theanine presents a strong substitute for conventional anxiolytic drugs. Its effectiveness in treating disorders like post-traumatic stress disorder, social anxiety disorder, and generalized anxiety disorder is being investigated in clinical trials.

Additionally, the potential applications of L-Theanine's cognitive enhancing qualities in a variety of academic and professional contexts are being investigated, especially in conjunction with caffeine. L-theanine-containing cognitive enhancement pills may grow in popularity as a way to promote mental clarity, attention, and alertness.

Given its neuroprotective properties, L-theanine may find use in the treatment and prevention of neurodegenerative disorders such as Parkinson's and Alzheimer's as research into the compound continues. Due to its antioxidant qualities, it can also be used to boost the immune system and promote cardiovascular health. This could help with the creation of nutraceuticals and dietary supplements.

L-theanine's medicinal potential is still being discovered despite continuous research, ranging from neuroprotection and sleep regulation to mental health and cognitive enhancement. In the sphere of health and well-being, more research and innovation are probably in store in the years to come, which should result in fresh perspectives and useful applications.

Testimonies And First-Hand Accounts

Personal experiences and testimonials might offer insightful information on the advantages and efficacy of L-theanine supplementation. Anecdotal evidence can provide some insight into how this amino acid affects people's lives, but it shouldn't take the place of scientific studies.

After taking L-Theanine pills, a lot of consumers have claimed to feel more at ease and relaxed. This is frequently explained by its capacity to stimulate the generation of alpha brain waves, which are linked to a relaxed, awake state. It is a well-liked option for people looking for a natural method to reduce anxiety and stress because users report feeling more focused and less worried.

Another feature that appears often in first-person narratives is the potential for L-theanine to improve cognitive performance. Users who use caffeine in particular report having better focus and mental clarity. Some people discover that L-theanine makes it easier for them to stay in a state of flow, which facilitates the completion of activities and creative activities.

L-theanine has received recognition for its capacity to enhance the quality of sleep in the domain of relaxation and sleep. Users have reported experiencing more uninterrupted and peaceful sleep, as well as a decrease in insomnia symptoms and even an improvement in lucid dreaming. The relaxing properties of this amino acid seem to extend into the evening, assisting people in unwinding and achieving restful sleep.

Applications In The Real World And Success Stories

Real-world uses for L-theanine include everything from improving performance to everyday living. Success stories demonstrate its adaptability and potential advantages in a range of fields.

Management of Stress and Anxiety: People who are struggling with the demands of contemporary life frequently use L-theanine for its ability to reduce stress. People who have successfully implemented it into their daily routines include professionals handling high-pressure professions, parents juggling work and home obligations, and students approaching exams. It's a useful tool for managing stress and anxiety because it can induce relaxation without making you sleepy.

Increasing Productivity: L-theanine and caffeine together are a well-liked option for people who want to improve their mental function. Success stories frequently feature professionals and students who report feeling more focused, alert, and able to concentrate for longer periods, which boosts output.

Good Sleep and Insomnia Relief: People who have trouble sleeping have commended the relaxing properties of L-theanine. People who have experienced relief from insomnia, sleep disorders, or restless nights are examples of success stories. It has aided individuals in getting a better night's sleep by encouraging relaxation and lowering anxiety.

Sports and Physical Performance: The effects of L-theanine on concentration and mental clarity can be used in sports and physical performance. It is now simpler for athletes to sustain top performance throughout the competition, according to athlete reports of increased focus and decreased performance anxiety.

Mood Regulation: L-theanine's ability to regulate mood is further demonstrated by success stories. People who experience emotional ups and downs have discovered that it can help them maintain a more stable and optimistic mindset, but it shouldn't be viewed as the only treatment for severe mood disorders.

Positive reviews and success stories of L-theanine supplements can be found in a wide range of applications, such as mood modulation, sports performance, cognitive enhancement, stress and anxiety management, and improved sleep.

Even though these first-hand accounts provide insightful information about the possible advantages of L-theanine, it's crucial to keep in mind that everyone reacts differently, and research into the whole spectrum of effects and mechanisms is still ongoing. Before beginning any new supplement regimen, always get medical advice, especially if you have underlying medical concerns or are currently taking other medications.

Professional Responses And Explanations

It's important to look into professional explanations and answers if you want to learn more about L-Theanine supplementation.

The mode of action of L-theanine, its interactions with other drugs, and the best dosage recommendations can all offer insightful information.

L-theanine's main mode of action is through its effects on neurotransmitters in the brain. Serotonin, a neurotransmitter linked to mood modulation, and GABA, an inhibitory neurotransmitter that encourages relaxation, are both increased by it. This can foster calmness while assisting in the reduction of stress and anxiety.

L-theanine is frequently combined with caffeine, especially in goods that aim to provide users with a steady, targeted energy boost. It is noteworthy that L-Theanine can counteract some of the adverse effects of caffeine, including jitters and elevated heart rate. Nootropic pills and "smart" drinks frequently contain this mix.

The ideal L-theanine dosage varies from person to person and is determined by the intended outcomes. A usual dosage of 100–200 mg is used to promote relaxation and reduce stress. It's usually advised to take 100 mg of L-theanine and 100 mg of caffeine in a 1:1 ratio when using the two together. Individual reactions could vary, though, so it's best to start with a smaller dose and raise it gradually as necessary.

Conclusion

L-theanine is a naturally occurring substance that shows promise in boosting sleep quality, lowering stress and anxiety, and encouraging relaxation. When taken as directed, it's generally safe to consume and won't lead to addiction.

Before beginning any new supplement routine, though, it's crucial to speak with a healthcare provider, particularly if you have underlying medical conditions or are taking medication. L-theanine and caffeine together are a popular combo for balanced energy and enhanced attention.

Individual responses may differ, as with any supplement, so it's best to keep an eye on the effects and change the dosage as needed to get the desired outcomes.

www.ingramcontent.com/pod-product-compliance
Lightning Source LLC
Chambersburg PA
CBHW060802260726
48660CB00002B/744